I0420359

What Every Girl Should Know

MARGARET SANGER

Copyright © 1916

ISBN: 978-1518749483

A. J. Cornell Publications

CONTENTS

1 INTRODUCTION

Students of vice, whether teachers, clergymen, social workers or physicians, have been laboring for years to find the cause and cure for vice, and especially for prostitution. They have failed so far to agree on either the cause or the cure, but it is interesting to know that upon one point they have been compelled to agree and that is that *ignorance of the sex functions* is one of the strongest forces that sends young girls into unclean living.

This, together with the knowledge of the rapidly increasing spread of venereal diseases and the realization of their subtle nature, has awakened us to the need of a saner and healthier attitude on the sex subject, and to the importance of *sex education* for boys and girls.

This need has shown itself so clearly that the question no longer seems to be, "Is there need of instruction?" but, "Who shall instruct?" Shall the mother or teacher instruct? When shall such instruction be given? In childhood, or in puberty? These are the points now under discussion.

To the writer the answer is simple. The mother is the logical person to teach the child as soon as questions arise, for it is to the mother that the child goes for information before he enters the schoolroom. If, therefore, the mother answers his questions truthfully and simply and satisfies his curiosity, she will find that the subject of sex ceases to be an isolated subject, and becomes a natural part of the child's general learning. A woman does not need to be a college graduate, with a special degree in the study of botany, before she can tell her child the beautiful truth of its birth. But she does need to clear her own mind of prudishness, and to understand that the procreative act is natural, clean and healthful; that all nature is beatified through it, and consequently that it is devoid of offensiveness.

If the mother can impress the child with the beauty and wonder and sacredness of the sex functions, she has taught it the first lesson, and the teacher can elaborate on those teachings as the child advances in school. All schools should teach the anatomy of the sex organs and their physiology, instead of teaching the human body in the neuter gender as has been done up to this time.

The whole object of teaching the child about reproduction through evolution is to clear its mind of any shame or mystery concerning its birth, and to impress it with the beauty, naturalness of procreation, in order to prepare it for the knowledge of puberty and marriage.

There must of necessity be special information for the pubescent boy and girl, for having arrived at the stage in their mental development they no longer take for granted what has been told of them by the parents, but are keen to form their own ideas and gather information independently. It is right, therefore, to give them the facts as science has found them.

There are workers and philanthropists who say there is too much stress put upon the subject of venereal diseases; that the young girl after learning or hearing of the dangers she is likely to encounter in the sexual relation, is afraid to marry and consequently lives a life unloved and alone.

"Your treatment of this subject is dangerous," said a very earnest social worker a few weeks ago. "Such knowledge will prevent our young girls from marrying."

To which I replied that my object in telling young girls the truth is for the definite purpose of preventing them from entering into sexual relations whether in marriage or out of it, without thinking and knowing. Better a thousand times to live alone and unloved than to be tied to a man who has robbed her of health or of the joy of motherhood, or welcoming the pains of motherhood, live in anxiety lest her sickly offspring be taken out of her life or grow up a chronic invalid.

I have more faith in the force of love. I believe that two people convinced that they love each other and desire to live together in marriage will talk as frankly of their own health and natures as they do today of house furnishings and salaries. Their love for each other will protect them from ill-health and disease, and prompt them to procure of their own accord a certificate of health if each has the right information and knowledge.

There are, however, different phases of nature other

than venereal disease, the knowledge of which binds and cements the love of two people. These are symptoms of a great social disorder.

Every girl should first understand herself: she should know her anatomy, including sex anatomy: she should know the epochs of a normal woman's life, and the unfoldment which each epoch brings: she should know the effect the emotions have on her acts, and finally she should know the fullness and richness of life when crowned by the flower of motherhood.

2 GIRLHOOD: PHYSICAL GROWTH

It has been said that the American girl between the ages of 12 and 13 is the most neglected girl in the world. Just why this is so, it is difficult to say, but I doubt whether she is alone in this neglect, for this is known as the *adolescent period*, and it is only within the last few years that this period has been at all considered, or its importance recognized in any part of the world.

The adolescent period is the time occupied between the ages of 12 and 22, when the physical development comes suddenly into prominence; when the mental faculties become independently active, and the sex of the individual strongly manifests itself. It is a period of the greatest importance to the girl herself, for her physical, mental and moral development during this time will have an important effect on her future life.

It is also a period of the greatest interest to the mother, provided there is sympathy, confidence and understanding between them. Too much importance cannot be attached to the necessity of an early confidence between the girl and her mother before this period arrives, for this will give the girl a sense of superiority, a poise, an understanding of herself and her nature. She will then be prepared for the changes taking place within herself, and consequently be practically immune from the influence of a bad environment, which otherwise might affect her in a way detrimental to her health and happiness. Up to this period there is very little manifestation of sex.

Fortunately we have come to recognize that healthy outdoor play is as good for the little girl as it is for the boy, and the ideas of our grandmothers' day—that boys were to play ball, ride horseback, swim, shoot, etc., while the girls, play was restricted to sedentary pursuits, such as sewing, doll playing, etc.—have been placed on the relic heap, and the girl of today keeps pace with her brother in physical freedom and activity.

With the passing of those ideas passed also our ideal of the delicate girl, with a cough, small waist and dainty appetite, and the girl physically strong and healthy, with a broader view of life, has taken her place.

About the age of 12 there comes a sudden change in the girl, her dresses are outgrown, her form assumes shape, her bust and limbs develop, and, in the words of Stanley Hall, "hips, thighs, limbs, shoulders, and arms round out into contours more or less beautiful, curves always pre-dominating over angles." Thus we come to realize that the little girl has left us.

The physical development is not alone in this work;

for the mental and moral instincts are developing so rapidly that it is difficult to understand this new and lovely creature who is neither the child of yesterday nor the woman of tomorrow.

There is often very little patience shown the adolescent girl, for neither parents nor teachers have been aware that this is a separate and distinct stage—this passing from childhood into womanhood—and as such must be recognized.

Let us first take the bony structure. It is a well-known fact that there is not sufficient lime salts in the system to complete the bony structure until the 25th year. The bones are not completely hardened, which is the reason that so many deformities have their foundation laid at this time.

The first and most noticeable change in the girl at this age is the increase of height, which begins at the 11th year and ends about the 15th. There are girls who begin earlier and continue to grow for several years after this age, but it is with the average we deal, and the growth after the age of 15 is not so perceptible.

Many girls show almost no other signs of womanly development until after this growth has ceased. The bones at this time are soft enough to yield to pressure (being cartilaginous), which makes the wearing of a corset especially dangerous, for the pressure on the ribs interferes with the development of the lungs and tuberculosis is more easily contracted. Corsets should not be worn before the 21st year if possible, and then very loosely, for tight lacing is more harmful at this age than a few years later.

The girl who scoffs at the idea of the Chinese women binding up their feet is doubtless ignorant of the knowledge that to bind up her own thoracic and pelvic structures—i.e., the chest, and abdominal portions of her body—in tight corsets is doing greater harm to her health and injury to her development than the binding of the feet could possibly do. As this rapid growth begins, the girl often finds it difficult to hold herself up straight, her shoulders become stooped, her head and neck are thrust forward in a most ungainly manner. As she becomes conscious of this, instead of correcting it, she is likely to slouch and assume the most awkward habits. Her arms seem longer to her; hands, legs and feet become new burdens to carry, and the desire to hide the hands behind the back, to fold the arms, to bend one knee in order to lessen the length of the body, and to lean on something while talking, are all signs of this consciousness.

With the invention of modern machinery and the monotony of specialized work in the mills and factories, it is natural that this should bring with it, if not entirely new diseases and deformities, at least a greater number than have heretofore been known. Consider the little children in the cotton mills, standing for long periods, with the weight of the body thrown on one foot—a position which causes curvature of the spine. Again, consider the young girls still in their "teens" bending over sewing machines from morning until night from year to year; their premium for this work is right-sided lateral curvature. Sitting with one leg crossed over the other as in sewing, carrying books under the arm to and from school, lifting and carrying heavy burdens, bundles, or small children, such as the abused and deformed "little mothers" spend their playtime in doing—all cause curvature of the spine.

Curvature is one of the most common deformities. Any position which throws the spinal column out of its natural line for any length of time is likely to produce it.

Regular exercise in the open air will do much to prevent this together with walking and dancing. If curvature is already noticeable, then it is best to get professional instructions and follow them closely.

Next to the rapid bony development, the changes in the heart and circulation are most noticeable. The heart grows more rapidly during the adolescent age than the arteries do, which increases the supply of blood in the arteries and causes general circulatory disturbance of which we see many outward signs such as blushing, nose bleed, headache, cold feet and hands, anemia, loss of appetite, or an appetite so capricious as to drive one frantic trying to satisfy it, for it jumps from ice cream soda to dill pickles, according to whim. Some of these symptoms require special attention, particularly in the case of the girl at school or in an office, who finds her work a great effort, tires easily, and becomes pale and nervous. Such a girl should spend as much time as possible in the open air, and build up on milk and eggs. Sometimes a simple iron tonic will do much to overcome these disturbances.

Pimples on the face are also very common at this period. Physicians assert that with cleanliness of the skin and regularity of the bowels, these symptoms will disappear without the aid of medicines or cosmetics. The above mentioned symptoms are of great annoyance to the adolescent girl, who is just developing pride in looking neat and keeping up the appearance of daintiness, and she goes to unending trouble to rid herself of facial blemishes, which in turn seem to grow worse and if tampered with leave ugly scars.

The nervous system also undergoes great changes at this age, and the growing girl is subject to various forms of nervous affections, stammering, jerking, restlessness, etc. These are symptoms which, if allowed to continue unattended, may develop into permanent disorders. In short, the adolescent girl needs constant watchfulness and attention.

3 GIRLHOOD: MENTAL DEVELOPMENT

The organs of sense are also awakened to activity in the adolescent girl. The sense of smell becomes extremely acute; offensive odors are *very* offensive, while pleasant ones are greatly enjoyed and desired. Thus we find perfumes used lavishly in girlhood, and alas! too often indiscriminately.

With the development of the other senses the sense of color is awakened. The girl who yesterday allowed her elders to choose clothing and colors for her at this time becomes most exacting in her own selection of ribbons and dresses. Sunsets and forests have become beautiful, and often the girl with artistic talent decides at this age to choose her life work. Laces, jewelry, trinkets, ribbons and shop windows become her world. Indeed, so great is her desire to possess ornaments that she has been known to resort to petty thievery, when unable to avail herself of the means to obtain them otherwise. Certain authorities, who have made vice and kindred subjects a study, assert that it is this great desire for trinkets, silk petticoats, etc., which induces girls to sell their bodies and enter prostitution. Such authorities fail to see the economic significance of these unsatisfied desires. There is something wrong with a system of society which allows its women to sell their bodies for such trifles, the desire for which is part of their natural development.

Is flesh and blood and the virtue of the mothers of the future so cheap in this land of plenty that it can be sacrificed for such passing whims? It is impossible to suppress that inherent and natural desire in the adolescent girl to adorn and beautify herself. She must and will do it.

The girl of wealth, of the so-called upper class, can beautify herself and adorn her body with the costliest jewels and fabrics. All eyes are upon her in admiration of her exquisite taste and attractive appearance. Yet this same manifestation in a working girl is condemned. Any attempt on the part of a working girl to give expression to the desire to be beautiful is considered "dangerous to her welfare"; is spoken of as her "awful desire for trinkets."

The women of wealth set certain standards for themselves and their class, but separate and distinct standards for the women of the working class. It is about time the reformers and philanthropists do something other than shake their heads over these bad "symptoms" shown by working girls.

A craving for beauty and pleasure, dancing, music, singing and laughter, an innate, hereditary desire to adorn and beautify herself, which comes down to her from primitive woman, together with a burning desire for and love of romance, characterize the adolescent girl and often remain with her far beyond the adolescent age.

When the imagination is thus aroused it is not unusual to learn that the young girl yields to it, tells strange tales about herself, and is, therefore, often accused of lying. But this and petty thievery disappear as reason and will power are developed.

The change of voice in a girl is not so distinct as in a boy, but the voice gradually becomes softer, fuller and of a more womanly pitch, though the change is quite unnoticeable while it occurs.

The hearing becomes keener, noises which a few months ago were considered a joke are now disturbing (such as father's loud sneeze). Music and singing have charms, which in childhood were unappreciated.

Parents and teachers who do not appreciate the change taking place within the girl at this period, have small patience with such doings, calling her "giddy" and "affected" when in reality it is all part of her development and can be guided and directed into beautiful channels. Together with her personal adornment comes interest in her surroundings. New and elaborate decorations furnish her bedroom, and toilet accessories become objects of pride. Primitive colors are displayed, largely in curtains, bed coverings, wall paper, etc., all of which explain the independent ego in the stage of transition.

There are many forms of disturbance which the girl suffers at this period, such as hysteria and insanity, which, however, we will not dwell upon here. Enough has been said on the subject to impress upon my readers the cause of these physical and mental disturbances, and to realize that special care and consideration should be given at this particular age of the girl.

The emotional nature also plays a most prominent part in the developing girl, and justice, I feel, would not be shown her here, unless we cover briefly this most interesting part of her nature. One of the strongest emotions which very few girls, passing from childhood into womanhood, escape is the religious awakening of one kind or another. It is said by some investigators that 80 percent of the conversions of women in the churches take place before the age of 20. From 30 to 40 years only a very small percentage occur—something like 1 or 2 percent.

It is also shown that more young girls join the church than boys. Some girls seem almost consumed by the desire to do good and be good in every thought and word and act, and have been known to go through various forms of self-punishment, such as fasting, sacrificing pleasure, etc. Again, others spend hours in absolute devotion to the neglect of health and studies. It is very easily seen why the church takes its "flock," while still in the adolescent period, for at no subsequent time is the girl's mind so plastic or impressionable. If the same girl who enters the convent at 18 years had waited until 22 she would very likely not have entered, for the mental changes are most intense from 16 to 18 years of age.

Another common emotional awakening of girlhood is the affections. In boys this awakening causes them to gather together in gangs. They follow the leader whom they greatly admire and obey. In girls it assumes a more simple form, the devotion to a girl friend of her own age, and the affection between them is deep and intense while it lasts. They tell their most private thoughts in secret to each other, dividing all honors, pleasures and gifts; they are almost inseparable, and I have known a girl whose affection was so deep for her "chum" that she wore mourning when the chum's father died.

Another form of affection which the girl of this age manifests is that for an older woman, often a teacher or neighbor. Parents sometimes look askance at this relation, and rightly so, for a friendship can be beneficial or harmful according to the character of the older woman. But with all these interests there is nothing so all-absorbing or so interesting the adolescent girl as *herself*. She has become conscious of *self*. Now she burns with ambition to go out into the world and do mighty things. She feels sure she will be a great singer, or a dancer, or, perhaps, an actress. Again, she feels she will write a wonderful book— about herself—or at least she will be the heroine. Or she will write a wonderful tragic play; or she will nurse on the battlefields and care for the sick and dying. These, together with thousands of other desires, burn in her mind, and can be increased or lessened according to the character of the books she reads. The literature placed in a girl's hands at this age has as great an influence on her thoughts and acts as her companions.

In early adolescence this self-consciousness manifests itself strongly. I mentioned previously the physical awkwardness of the girl. With this comes the blushing, and giggling, which are all signs that she is conscious of that inner self of the ego.

It is at this stage when the mother tries to explain what the menstrual period means to the girl that she is met with an icy indifference. She refuses to talk on this subject, or any thing pertaining to the sex subject, because she has just become conscious of her sex, and everything connected with it seems offensively personal.

She most likely has received her sexual information from some one else, and the mother is astonished at the stubborn silence on the part of her daughter. She fails to realize that some one else has that confidence which belongs to her and which she should have gained many years earlier. There is a strong tie between the adolescent girl and her sexual informant. The influence of an older girl over a younger, between whom there are confidences regarding sex is surprisingly great. The mind at this age is very susceptible to influences of any kind, and the ideals instilled into a girl's mind are of paramount importance.

These are only a few of the disturbances of the adolescent girl. But they are sufficient for us to know that at the bottom of all these disturbances is the mysterious influence of sex, gradually unfolding itself and finally claiming its own.

At the time these emotions are in full sway along comes a newer and deeper one. The boy with whom she has played for the past several years, run races, played house, ball and games, one day looks into her eyes—and something happens.

Perhaps that look was accompanied by a pull at her hair, a pinch on her arm, or a hit with an apple core, but the glance was one which awakened within her a new instinct; the consciousness of sex, and upon her horizon man appears.

Those who have investigated boy and girl love affairs seem to be of the opinion that they are invariably of short duration. Out of 100 high school girls interrogated, two had married while at school, and one of these had received a divorce shortly after. This goes to prove that the boy a girl is willing to elope with, or even starve for at 18, is quite forgotten at the age of 25.

Thousands of girls marry between the ages of 19 and 20—the years when they are developing in body, mind and character. They are at a loss to understand themselves, because they are ignorant of the fact that the wonderful instinct of sex is making itself felt. For thousands of years this instinct has been in the germ of life. When they have reached that age nature is preparing them to proclaim its right, to perform their natural functions, to propagate.

4 PUBERTY: GENERAL ORGANS, UTERUS, OVARIES, ETC.

Puberty is the age at which the girl or boy becomes capable of reproduction. Writers differ in the use of the word. Many use it to denote the whole period of time during which the procreative ability continues which is usually from the 14th to the 45th year. There are still other uses of the word, but we will use it as the age when the boy or girl becomes sexually matured or ripe, the first indication of which is the menstrual flow in the girl and seminal emissions in the boy.

This age of puberty is celebrated by initiations among savage peoples, mostly for the purpose of trying the powers of endurance in the boy or girl. The boy is taken away among strange tribes, is subjected to the greatest physical pain and hardship, and among some tribes is circumcised. The girl is often subjected to a vaginal incision and should she cry out or show any sign of suffering she is disgraced among the women of her tribe and promptly expelled from the settlement. In Ellis' *Psychology of Sex* the author relates of the Yuman Indians of California how the girls prepare for marriage at the first sign of menstruation by being wrapped in blankets and placed in a warm pit for four days and nights. The old women of the tribe dance about them and sing constantly; they give away coin, cloth and wheat to teach the girls generosity, and sow wild seeds broadcast over the girls to cause them to be prolific. These and various other initiations are practiced by nearly all savage tribes. The boys and girls receive their sex knowledge at this time, and are instructed in the duties of married life.

The girls are fully informed of the menstruation. It has been said the knowledge of sexual relations is openly discussed and naturally taught; that therefore, it has no glamour for men, and that in consequence the women of these tribes are virtuous.

Perhaps you will wonder what bearing all this has on *What Every Girl Should Know*. I relate it only to show that the savages have recognized the importance of plain sexual talks to their young for ages, while civilization is still hiding itself under the black pall of prudery.

When we speak of puberty it is necessary to have some knowledge of the organs of reproduction and their structure. So far the physiology taught in the public schools has not treated of these organs. In order to get books on this subject a girl is met with the question: "Are you a nurse or physician?" If not, the books are denied her. Consequently the average girl is kept in ignorance of the function of these organs, and is at a loss to know where to go for clean information. It is necessary, therefore, to give this information here, without mincing words, if there is any benefit to be derived from the following chapters. It is very simple for the girl to learn the correct names of these organs and call them by such names. They are the *ovaries, fallopian tubes, uterus, vagina* and *breasts.* The breasts were not always classed as reproductive organs, but later writers recognize their relation to them, and as such they are now included.

Let us first take the ovaries, which are two small glands about the size and shape of an almond, placed one at each side of the extreme lower part of the woman's abdomen. They are imbedded in large muscles which also help to hold the uterus (the womb) in place. Inside the ovaries are thousands of little eggs called ovules, which have been there since the birth of the girl. The work of the ovary is to develop and mature these eggs, and send them on to be fertilized. At the time of puberty, these eggs are all in different stages of development. Those in the center of the ovary ripen first and burst through the outer cover of the ovary (which is like a capsule and at the time of menstruation becomes swollen and congested). The ovule is caught by the fringy ends of the fallopian tubes, which are in a constant lashing motion, which motion sends the egg through the tube to the uterus.

The fallopian tubes join the ovaries to the upper and outer angle of the uterus. Sometimes the sperm cell from the male comes up into the tube to meet the egg and it is fertilized here, but this is not the nest nature has prepared for the egg's development, and unless it returns into the uterus it causes serious trouble and an operation is necessary. Impregnation in the tube is very rare, but it is possible.

The uterus, often spoken of as the womb, is a hollow muscular organ into which the egg comes from the tubes to be fertilized. After fertilization it remains here, is nourished and developed until it can develop no more. Then it is thrown out by the contraction of the muscles, which process we call the birth of the child. The uterus is about three inches long, its shape is like a pear with the small end downward. It is not fastened to any of the bony parts, but is held in place by the ligaments and muscles, which also allow it to move with different movements of the body. One of the most interesting features about the uterus which is so small in its cavity is that it can attach to accommodate the growing child within it to the length of nineteen to twenty-one inches. This is because it is one and one-half inches thick and composed of layers of muscles which are tough and yet elastic. At the upper side of the uterus are the openings into the fallopian tubes. At the small end of uterus is another opening leading into the vagina. It is through this opening the sperm of the male comes in order to fertilize the egg. Thus you can readily see the uterus is the nest or cradle where the egg is to live until it becomes strong enough to subsist on other nourishment.

The vagina is a muscular tube-like passage which extends from the small part of the uterus (called the neck) to the outer surface of the body where its opening is usually partly closed in virgins by a thin membrane or film known as the *hymen*. The walls of the vagina are also very thick and elastic. This is sometimes called the birth canal. The hymen was for years a subject for discussion in the professional world among physicians. In my talks to girls I find it a subject of great interest and often anxiety to many of them, for the average girl seems possessed with the old idea that the presence of the hymen is necessary to marital happiness. The time was not long ago when its absence was considered cause for serious discord between husband and wife, and I have been told that under the old law its absence was sufficient ground for divorce.

Fortunately, modern science has thrown some light on this subject and disproved the theory that its absence was necessarily due to a woman's having had sexual relations. There are cases on record of women who have lived four and five years in prostitution who were found with perfectly preserved hymen. It is important to know that it differs in size and shape in women. Also, that in some women it has been entirely absent since birth. It can be destroyed by accident or injured by operations, or examinations where the physician did not use the greatest care. In some women it is easily destroyed; in others it is more difficult. It is not at all uncommon for a physician to find the hymen unruptured when he comes to deliver the firstborn child. All of which goes to prove that neither its presence nor its absence is necessarily the sign of virginity.

5 PUBERTY: MENSTRUATION AND ITS DISORDERS

Beginning with puberty the eggs from the ovary are expelled as they ripen or mature. This process is called *ovulation* and occurs about every twenty-eight days. It is closely related to menstruation but it is not menstruation as you will soon learn.

Some writers say the egg is expelled at other times than at the menstrual periods; another writer asserts that one passes every six hours, alternating male and female. There are many views and ideas on the subject of ovulation, but I will tell you of the most generally accepted theory, that the egg is expelled from the ovary every twenty-eight days.

When the eggs ripens, the ovary discharges it and sends it on to find its way through the tubes to the uterus. Here we find the blood supply of the uterus greatly increased in preparation for the egg. We find the inner lining of the uterus becomes very soft and smooth so that the egg can very easily find a place in which to lodge itself until it becomes fertilized. We also find that the cells swell and multiply, all in preparation to welcome and nourish the incoming egg or ovum. If the egg is fertilized by the male, it then remains in the uterus to develop. If not, it is thrown out, together with all the preparation made to receive it. The cells burst and discharge their contents; the mucus blood, cells and all come away in what is called the *menstrual flow*.

At one time woman was thought to be the only creature which menstruated. But science now tells us that all warm blooded animals which walk erect menstruate. The discharge is chiefly due to the position which in standing upright throws the large part of the uterus higher than the neck. In animals, such as dogs, cats, etc., the same process goes on, but the position of these animals keeps the large part of the uterus lower than the small part, where the blood is retained and then reabsorbed into the system.

This process goes on every four weeks in girls after they reach the age of puberty and continues at regular periods as long as the egg is not fertilized until the reproductive age is over, which is usually between the 45th and 50th year. If, however, the egg is fertilized the menstrual flow ceases and this blood supply goes to nourish the new life in the uterus. It does not appear again until after the birth of the child, and usually ceases while the child depends on the milk from the mammal glands.

The age at which this process (menstruation) first

takes place in girls differs in individuals. Climate has some effect upon it, for girls in warm or Southern climates mature earlier than in colder places. In this climate the average girl reaches puberty at 14 years of age. Some have been known to reach it as early as the 11th and others not until the 18th year, in all in the same place and yet normal and healthy, which shows there is no reason for anxiety if the girl does not menstruate at 14, provided she is developing normally and is in good health. During the first few years after its appearances the periods are likely to be irregular. This is because the sexual organs are not fully developed. Often the period does not occur after the first time for three, five, eight months, and sometimes a year. This irregularity continues for two or three years. Cases of girls coming from Europe have been known where the period was perfectly established over there, but after arriving in this climate the menstrual flow did not occur again for a year and over. Usually this irregularity lasts only a few months, and once it has become regular, there should be no worry over its arrival a day or two earlier or later.

The length of time the period lasts differs in women also. The average length of time is four or five days, yet there are women in which it lasts fully a week, and others but a few hours. The length of time should not be of as much concern as the amount of discharge which is expelled each time. It is, of course, difficult to estimate this, but physicians claim that more than three protectives in twenty-four hours should not be used. In all women the flow is more profuse during the first two days.

The care of the health should receive more attention during the first two days than is usually given it. To the girl who has to work from early morning until late at night, these two days are unusually hard on her nerves and on her general health, and I regret that I have no new message for her to help lighten the burden, which under the present atrocious industrial system makes it so hard for her.

Physicians say there should be no need of interrupting the regular routine of the day at this time more than any other. There are a few strong women to whom this period makes no difference, but the average girl in this country spends two days of pain and discomfort. Out of 1,000 girls questioned, only 16 percent were entirely free from pain, which proves that the time has come for women to cease being ashamed of this function, and insisting upon at least one day's rest at the expense of her employer. Some of the old biblical ideas instilling into the man's mind that a woman is unclean at this time has been the cause of much hardship and many sneers endured by a woman during these periods. The consequence has been that she will bear the most intense pain rather than allow the men working with her to suspect that she is menstruating. It is all nonsense and wrong, and it is time women should band together in one great sisterhood to protect one another from being slowly drained and exhausted of their powers of motherhood for the benefit of their exploiters. Women who belong to unions should demand that this day be given them and their sisters. Girls continue to suffer pains in the abdomen and back, pains running down the limbs, headache, often nausea, besides being nervous and irritable, yet hang on a strap in an overcrowded street car, stand or sit all day in the shop or at the machine and utter no protest. They know, too, they are not alone in this suffering, for they see about them day after day hundreds of other women enduring the same pain, yet they remain silent.

How long will you endure this, working women?

There is one thing to remember, that the greatest strain comes on the nervous system at this period. One of the best ways to assist in building up the nerve strength is in sleep and rest and for the girl who dares not remain away from the shop fearing to lose her "job" the next best thing is to get to bed early, for there is nothing that builds up the exhausted nerves like sleep. Fortunately, the girl at school has some consideration shown her at this time, and it is well that this is so, for until the period becomes established there is special danger of overdoing in schoolwork, which often causes St. Vitus dance and other nervous disorders.

I believe firmly in the regular warm tub bath, or cold sponge followed by a good rubbing all over the body at this time, together with nine or ten hours' sleep, and light nourishing food without stimulant. If the bowels are active, it often lessens the pain considerably, and it is very important that every girl attend to this if she has any regard for her health. There are a few abnormalities of the menstrual function which I will not take the space to state here. Before leaving the subject, I wish to impress upon the reader that most abnormalities, such as too little or too much flow, or very great exhausting pain are usually caused, not by any diseases of the generative organs, but more often a disturbance of the general health, which can often be treated and cured by building up the system.

6 SEXUAL IMPULSE: MASTURBATION

The sexual impulse is the strongest force in all living creatures. It is this that animates the struggle for existence; it is this that attracts and unites two beings, that they may reproduce their kind; it is this that inspires man to the highest and noblest thoughts; it is this also that inspires man to all endeavors and achievements, to all art and poetry; this impulse is the creative instinct which dominates all living things and without which life must die. If, then, this force, this impulse plays so strong a part in our lives, is it not necessary that we know something of it?

At the time of puberty there comes both to boys and girls two impulses—one, the desire to touch and caress; to come in contact with, to write and to speak to an individual of the opposite sex. This impulse is much stronger in girls than in boys. The other is the impulse that impels the individual to discharge the accumulation of ripe sex cells, and relieve himself of the nervous tension which this accumulation produces. This latter impulse is stronger in boys than in girls. One writer states that this is an unconscious desire for relief from physical congestion, not differing greatly from the sense of relief which the emptying of the bladder or rectum produces.

These two impulses together constitute the Sexual Impulse, and this constitutes the foundation upon which love, the greatest of all emotions, is based.

At the time of puberty, the first manifestations of sexual maturity in the girl is the appearance of the menstrual flow. But also at puberty there comes the sexual impulse, which evidences itself during sleep, in a filmy substance dropping from the mouth of the uterus. This "demunescense" does not appear very often in young girls, but later in life when sex instinct becomes stronger it occurs during sleep, especially in young widows, or women having experienced sexual relations. They are, however, seldom aware of its taking place; consequently, it has not the danger which it presents to the boy.

In the chapter on puberty, we discussed only the girl at puberty, but here it is necessary to understand that during puberty many changes take place in the boy, such as change of voice, the growth of hair on various parts of the body, and most important, the discharge of the sexual fluid commonly known as seminal emissions. This latter symptom appears in every normal healthy boy on reaching the age of puberty, but unlike the menstrual period which occurs at a stated period in girls, the seminal emissions do not depend upon a special period; they occur at different times, usually twice a month. This expulsion is considered perfectly normal, and is not a sign of physical or sexual weakness, but a sign that a surplus accumulation of ripe sex cells are present and have come to their full development and overflow. Nature takes care of this and uses all of this life giving fluid according to the needs of the individual, casting off the surplus.

It is this symptom that alarms young boys at puberty. It is this overflow which enables quack doctors to play upon the innocent and ignorant boy, telling him that it is an indication of weakness. And it is also this—as the result of telling older boys about it—that leads boys to houses of prostitution; for they are told by their ignorant advisers that they must have sexual relations or endanger their sexual capacity.

It is also this overflow which, occurring in sleep, awakens the boy, and he is conscious of what has occurred; he is conscious also of a pleasurable sensation which this sense of relief produces, and unless warned against it he will try at some later time to bring on this relief by friction or mechanical means, which is known as masturbation—often called self-abuse. The age of puberty is one of the periods in an individual's life in which it is easiest to acquire this habit, in girls as well as in boys, although the girl may not be conscious of any sensation, through the accumulation of the "demunescense." Yet there is the same nervous tension that exists in boys, due to congestion of the now fully developed genital organs, perhaps slighter in intensity, but it is there and becomes conscious of it.

In talking to older girls about sex, menstruation, etc., she is often led into the habit of masturbation. Cases have been known where children formed this habit in infancy almost, through the ignorance of nurses or even mothers, who, not aware of consequences, have kept babies from crying by gently patting or rubbing the sexual parts. It may be caused also by uncleanliness, itching, tight clothing, etc.

When the habit is formed in very small children, it can be exercised in the very presence of the parents, but they being ignorant of the habit itself, or the consequences, interpret the actions as "baby ways." Again, the habit is formed upon entering school. It is said no school is free from it; and it is a fact that no institution today is free from pupils who practice masturbation.

In public schools are found groups of perverted boys and girls whose depraved ideas sooner or later permeate the place. A recent issue of a conservative woman's journal says: "In absolute filth of conversation nothing could quite equal the talk of boys and girls during recess in our schools. What is still worse is that the child is generally instructed in masturbation, prostitution and sometimes sexual perversity."

This subject of masturbation is at present under discussion from many points of view among the medical profession; some claiming, that, as with venereal diseases, we lay too much stress on the matter, and exaggerate the harm done to the individual by it. One writer plainly states that it is of such common practice that out of a hundred young men and women, ninety-nine are addicted to it, and the hundredth one is lying. Another says that out of a hundred men and women arriving at the age of 25, ninety-nine have practiced it at some time.

Moreover, it is said to be practiced by people of nearly every race on the globe, and even by animals when sexually aroused and their mates are not near. By these examples such writers would try to prove that because ninety-nine people out of one hundred are not in insane asylums the practice cannot be as harmful as is stated by others to be.

Let us take a sane and logical view of this subject and arrive at a decided conclusion.

In children before they have reached the age of puberty, prior to the development of the sexual organs, it stands to reason that to abuse these organs before they are strong enough to be exercised must weaken them for their natural functions. Again, masturbation unlike the sexual act, can be practiced individually and at all times and nearly anywhere. This gives the individual unlimited opportunity for indulgence, and consequently drains and exhausts the system of the vitality necessary for full development.

In the boy or girl past puberty we find one of the most dangerous forms of masturbation, i.e., mental masturbation, which consist of forming mental pictures, or thinking of obscene or voluptuous pictures. This form is considered especially harmful to the brain, for the habit becomes so fixed that it is almost impossible to free the thoughts from lustful pictures. Every girl should guard against the man who invariably turns a word or sentence into a lustful, or commonly termed, "smutty" channel, for nine times out of ten he is a mental masturbator.

Perhaps the greatest physical danger to the chronic masturbator is the inability to perform the sexual act naturally. The strong physical irritants which are used are likely to produce catarrhal disease of these organs in both sexes, producing such irritating sensations that relief is demanded, and this can be obtained only by repeating the habit, and so it continues. The individual promises himself over and over again after such exercises to overcome the habit, but his will power gradually becomes destroyed and the impulse continues. He knows and intuitively feels such practice degrades him and destroys his character; he feels he is losing control of himself, and also realizes that his health, especially his nervous system, is being undermined.

In my personal experience as a trained nurse while attending persons afflicted with various and often revolting diseases, no matter what their ailments, I never found any one so repulsive as the chronic masturbator.

It would not be difficult to fill page upon page of heart-rending confessions made by young girls, whose lives were blighted by this pernicious habit, always begun so innocently.

Before closing this subject, however, I want to tell of a case of an 8-year-old boy I attended during an attack of measles. I found he was shy and unresponsive, and at times very nervous and irritable, with a strong liking to be alone. I observed him closely for a few days and reported the results of my observation to the attending physician.

He was convinced of their truth, that the little fellow was masturbating. The physician assigned to me the task of talking to the child, who acknowledged that he was "touching" himself and had been ever since he could remember. The little fellow's mother had died when he was in infancy, leaving beside himself a brother a year older with whom he slept. I explained to him the danger as well as I could and the result was that I was awakened in the night by whisperings and found the little fellow asking the older brother to tie his hands to the bedpost. This the older brother did with a handkerchief, and the child went to sleep in this way every night during the few weeks I was attending him. The first few nights he was awake practically all of the time struggling to overcome this habit, which he finally overcame completely.

At puberty every boy and girl should be taught these dangers and temptations and also how to avoid them, by keeping active, mentally and physically, going to bed only when sleepy, avoiding intoxicating drinks and stimulants.

7 SEXUAL IMPULSE: SEXUAL IMPULSE IN ANIMALS, IN MEN; ITS SIGNIFICANCE IN LOVE

In the previous chapter we learned that the sexual impulse is a combination of the two impulses, the one which impels the discharge of ripe sex cells, strongest in the boy, and the other which impels the individual to touch or caress an individual of the opposite sex, strongest in the girl.

Every girl has in mind an ideal man. This ideal begins to form sometime in the early adolescent age. He is usually distinct in her mind as to his physical qualities, such as dark or light hair, or brown or blue eyes. He is always a certain physical type, and often remains an ideal to her through life. At the forming period of the type she will be attracted toward many men who seem to answer the ideal type, but as she reads and develops through the various stages of the adolescent period, the ideal changes and grows with her. As she reaches the romantic stage the ideal must be brave, daring, courteous. If she is inclined toward out-door sports he must be athletic. And so it goes on until the twenty-third year, when the average girl has a fairly settled idea of the man who would suit her as a mate through life.

When the sexual impulse makes itself felt strongly in the adolescent boy or girl, they, feeling satisfied with the physical beauty and perfection of the other, marry, they are unconscious that the incentive to love when based on physical attraction alone is soon destroyed. For sickness, poverty or disease will affect even the most seemingly perfect physical attraction.

Let us not confuse the sexual impulse with love, for it alone is not love, but merely a necessary quality for the growth of love.

No sexual attraction or impulse is the foundation of the beautiful emotion of love. Upon this is built respect, self-control, sympathy, unity of purpose, many common tastes and desires, building up and up until this real love unites two individuals as one being, one life. Then it becomes the strongest and purest emotion of which the human soul is capable.

There is no doubt that the natural aim of the sexual impulse is the sexual act, yet when the impulse is strongest and followed by the sexual act without love or any of the relative instincts which go to make up love, the relations are invariably followed by a feeling of disgust. Respect for each other and for one's self is a primary essential to this intimate relation.

In plant and animal life the reproductive cell of the male is the active seeker of the passive female cell, imbued with the instinct to chase and bodily capture the female cell for the purpose of reproduction.

This instinct man, as he is today, has inherited, and, as with the lower forms of life, the senses are intensely involved. It is kept alive by the sense of sight, sound and smell, and reaches its highest development through the sense of touch. It is heightened by touching smooth and soft surfaces—which is said to account for the pleasure of kissing.

Earlier I spoke of the desire to touch being stronger in girls than in boys. This desire leads a girl to kiss and fondle a man without any conscious desire for the sexual act; whereas in the man, to be touched and caressed by the girl for whom he has a sexual attraction, stimulates the accumulation of sex cells, and the desire for the sexual act becomes paramount in his mind. Many a young girl bubbling over with the joy of living, innocent of any serious consequences, is oft-times misjudged by men on account of these natural actions. But she soon puts on her armor of defense, and stifles and represses any outbursts of affection.

Society, too, condemns the natural expression of Woman's emotion, save under certain prescribed conditions. In consequence of this, women suppress their maternal desires and today direct this great force into other channels, participating in the bigger and broader movements and activities in which they are active today.

This is one reason why the type of the so-called "old maid," so characteristic of the generation past, has disappeared. These great maternal powers are being used up in the activities of modern life. Instead of allowing it to remain dormant and make her odd and whimsical, the modern Woman turns her sexual impulse into a big directing force.

That the male creature is the pursuer of the female in all forms of life, there is no question, but that the female has the choice of selection and uses fine discrimination in her choice, cannot be denied either. This instinct of selection seems to lie dormant in women of today, for at puberty nature calls to every girl to make a selection suitable to her nature. Yet few girls follow this instinct on account of the specter of economic insecurity which looms up before them. Instead of asking themselves: "Are we matable and sympathetic?" they ask: "Shall we have enough food, clothing and shelter?"

Indeed, girls, this system increases our degradation, and places us in ideals lower than the animals. All over the civilized world today girls are being given and taken in marriage with but one purpose in view; to be well supported by the man who takes her. She does not concern herself with the man's physical condition: his hereditary taints, the cleanliness of his mind or past life, nor with the future race.

There will no doubt be a great change in Woman's attitude on this subject in the next few years. When women gain their economic freedom they will cease being playthings and utilities for men, but will assert themselves and choose the father of their offspring. As Bernard Shaw tells of her in one of his greatest plays, she will hunt down her ideal in order to produce the Superman.

There seems to be a general tendency on the part of the Woman who is demanding political freedom, to demand sexual freedom also. When a girl reaches the age nearing thirty her natural development tends toward sexual freedom. It seems as though nature, knowing the time of reproduction is drawing to a close, calls with all the fury of her strength to complete its development and procreate.

It is at this age where physicians claim a Woman awakens to the sexual desire, and it is at this age that women seek affection, or gratification with a "lover." To her there is nothing to say; she is mature, developed and can judge for herself where best her happiness lies.

But to the young girl at the age of say twenty, or even younger, immature, mentally undeveloped, there is something she should know, and that is that every physical impulse, every sensual feeling, every lustful desire will come to her whitewashed with the sacred word *love*.

Neither the boy nor the girl knows the difference between the sexual impulse and love. A boys meets a girl, he feels a great attraction for her, he feels the sexual impulse throbbing within him, he is full of this life giving current he feels it throughout his being, he walks lighter and straighter, he feels it in his voice, in his laughter, he grows tenderer within himself, and to women. He feels all this and is sure it is a love that will never die. If there is an attraction on the girl's part there is no difficulty in persuading her that this feeling IS love.

But it is not love; it is the creative force of sexual impulse scattered through his being and the sexual act brings it to its climax.

If motherhood comes to the girl through this relation, she has developed and the experience has enriched her life. But today the girl has an idea she has escaped the greatest disgrace when she has avoided motherhood. If the relation was based on physical attraction, a few abortions and the monotony of every day life soon remove this, and the man goes elsewhere in search of this wonderful sensation which he felt at first, but did not know how to keep or how to use.

The girl, however, has become a new being, sexually awakened and conscious of it. But ignorant of the use of the forces she possesses, she plunges forth blindly, with social and economic forces against her, and prostitution beckoning at every turn. So she soon passes with the crowd on the road to the Easiest Way. This is the story of thousands of young girls living in prostitution.

Women should know that the creative instinct does not need to be expended entirely on the propagation of the race. Though the sex cells are placed in a part of the anatomy for the essential purpose of easily expelling them into the female for the purpose of reproduction there are other elements in the sexual fluid which are the essence of blood, nerve, brain and muscle. When redirected into the building and strengthening of these we find men or women of the greatest endurance and greatest magnetic power. A girl can waste her creative powers by brooding over a love affair to the extent of exhausting her system, with results not unlike the effects of masturbation and debauchery.

Of course the sexual impulse is natural. It is natural in animals, degenerates, and in normal man. But in man it is mixed with other essentials which, together, are termed love. These essentials are derived from man's power of reasoning by which he is known as a higher species and through which he differs from the animals.

When man emerged from the jungle and stood upright on his hind legs, the shape of his head and his face changed from the long jaw and flat head of the animal to the flat face and high head of the man. All progress from that time forward was made along mental lines. According to the universal law then in existence he should have been limited to a geographical area and killed by the extreme heat or cold or starved for one kind of food if it were not obtained, but against all these he fought, because he became endowed with such attributes as reason, knowledge and will-power. Instead of using his creative powers solely in hunting food and reproducing his species, he used this force in making plans for his self-preservation. He built rafts and boats to cross rivers and streams, he devised methods of clothing himself against extreme heat and cold and discovered various ways of preparing food for different climates suitable for his various needs. In other words he conserved his creative force and redirected it into channels which have resulted in giving him precedence over all other living creatures. For man has developed a conscious mind which asserts itself by reasoning, which in turn has developed his brain-power.

It is said a fish as large as a man has a brain no larger than the kernel of an almond. In all fish and reptiles where there is no great brain development, there is also no conscious sexual control. The lower down in the scale of human development we go the less sexual control we find. It is said that the aboriginal Australian, the lowest known species of the human family, just a step higher than the chimpanzee in brain development, has so little sexual control that police authority alone prevents him from obtaining sexual satisfaction on the streets. According to one writer, the rapist has just enough brain development to raise him above the animal, but like the animal, when in heat knows no law except nature which impels him to procreate whatever the result. Every normal man and Woman has the power to control and direct his sexual impulse. Men and women who have it in control and constantly use their brain cells in thinking deeply, are never sensual.

It is well to understand that the natural aim of the sexual impulse is the sexual act and the natural aim of the sexual act is reproduction, though it does not always result in this. It is possible for conception to take place without love, it is even possible that there is no conscious knowledge to procreate before or during the act, yet this does not disprove the fact that nature has designed it for the purpose of reproduction, no matter what uses man has put it to today. This subject of procreation we shall discuss next.

Every girl should know that to hold in check the sexual impulse; to absorb this power into the system until there is a freely conscious sympathy, a confidence and respect between her and her ideal; that this will go toward building up the sexual impulse and will make the purest, strongest and most sacred passion of adult life, compared to which all other passions pale into insignificance.

8 REPRODUCTION: GROWTH OF THE LIFE CELL IN THE UTERUS

In teaching children or young persons the process of reproduction one of the cleanest, most natural and beautiful methods of doing this is to tell them the process which goes on in the various forms of life in the flower, fish, frog, bird and animal, leading up to the highest and most complex of all living creatures—man.

They watched the butterfly and bee carry a load of pollen from the father buttercup to fertilize the seeds within the mother flower. They watched Mr. and Mrs. Frog awaken from their long winter nap, and stirred by the life-giving impulse within them, start for the breeding pond. They watched Father Thrush win his mate and patiently stand guard over her during the tedious hatching days. They were told and saw that the that the flowers depended upon outside forces to bring the pollen from the male to the female to fertilize the seeds before the seeds could grow. They were taught that the mother fish lays her eggs in the water first and that the father fish, unlike the flowers, being able to move about, carries the pollen (which is now a fluid) to the seeds himself. They were told that Father Frog, being a higher creature, fertilized the eggs before they reached the water, and Father Thrush being still higher in the scale fertilized the eggs before they left the mother's body. That the higher the species was, the greater the care required to preserve that species.

In this way the mind is prepared for the information which should follow.

The girl at puberty should be taught this process and something of what goes on within the womb after the ovum has been fertilized. She should know that all organic life is the result of a simple cell; that man is a community of cells, banded together and depending upon each cell to carry on its work, for the benefit of the whole.

Let us first, then, get an idea of a cell and what it is and what it does. A cell is a tiny portion of living matter having in its center a spot or nucleus which represents the point of germination; it is separated from its sister cells by partitions of cell membrane.

A simple cell is formed by the fusion of two germ cells when they meet to exchange nuclear elements. After this fusion they are able to proceed with fission which means splitting into parts and it is the subsequent cellular growth of the fused germ cell that constitutes reproduction.

There are two kinds of reproductive cells, the ova in the female and the spermatozoa in the male.

When the sexual act takes place, there is deposited into the vagina a secretion know as semen. According to Sutkowsky, each deposit or ejaculation contains 50,000,000 of spermatozoa.

About the same time in the act there occurs in the female spasmodic contractions of the muscles of the uterus which draws in a small amount of the sperm which the male has left there.

The sperm cell of the male under the microscope shows that it contains both a head and a tail.

The tail enables it to move and advance with a tad-pole-like motion toward the ovum.

As in the lower forms of life, the male cell has within it the instinct to chase and capture the female cell. Consequently, it does not depend upon the uterine contractions of the female to enable it to reach the ovum for fertilization. The vagina being a corrugated or wrinkled tube, hides and secretes the sperm cell for days, unless it is removed with water or killed by poison.

When, however, the sperm comes near the ovum it is drawn to it as to a magnet.

The ovum being carefully protected by nature within the ovaries, leaves its sister cells and travels alone. The sperm cell, however, having more dangerous paths to travel, must provide against the uncertainty of doing its great work by going in numbers, though it takes but one single cell to produce human life.

A number of the male cells go to meet the ovum, but

only one enters it. Almost at the moment the head enters the ovum it becomes completely absorbed by the ovum and all trace of it is lost.

This union of the two cells is called *fertilization, fecundation, impregnation,* or *conception.* Any of these terms may be used. This union usually takes place in the tube, but the fertilized egg does not remain there; it wanders along and finds its way into the uterus.

Now that the ovum has been fertilized, it readily becomes attached to the soft lining of the uterus which has been specially prepared to receive it. No menstruation occurs. The woman is now *pregnant.* A new being is created, and marvelous changes will now take place within the tiny cell clinging so weakly to the lining of the uterus. At this time the ovum is so small it can scarcely be seen by the naked eye, but in two weeks it has grown to the size of a pea, in four weeks to the size of a walnut and in eight weeks to the size of a lemon. At this time it is three inches long and is completely formed, the head being much larger in proportion to the rest of its body. What has happened to the ovum in these few weeks is briefly this: Immediately after fertilization the ovum begins to divide into sections or lobes, into 3, 4, 8, 16, 32, etc.—cells until they are almost countless. Each cell splits in the middle of the nucleus, forming two complete new cells and so on.

The next stage is represented by this mass of cells forming themselves into a shape like a hollow ball. The third stage is the meeting of the two layers of cells, as if the bell had collapsed, and these two layers meet and unite as one, stretch and flatten out.

After this stage things become more complicated, new organs begin to develop, spine marks for the backbone and intestinal canal show themselves as do the bony and muscular structure of the skeleton.

A slight pulsation is observed, showing the development of the heart. The head fold is formed by a gradual bending of the spinal column at the front end of the ovum, which we will now call the *embryo*. There are also formed at this time processes which soon become arms and legs, there is a furrow for the face; pits for the eyes; all of which has happened in less than four weeks.

From this time forward development is rapid, the bones, which up to this time have been soft matter, grow harder, and all organs which were only outlined now become definitely formed. At the end of the fourth month it has grown to its natural shape. The remaining months it increases in size and gains strength. The uterus becomes enlarged, rises out of the pelvis and occupies the abdominal cavity. It takes forty weeks or 280 days to complete the growth of the human embryo, although the time may be two weeks more or less and yet be normal.

Let us see how the child has been fed all this time. When the ovum is fertilized and up to the eighth week it is fed by delicate branched threads which form a covering for it. These threads are called *villa*, and dip into the uterine surface for nourishment, from the mother to supply the embryo.

About the eighth week these villa have grown greatly intertwined into a mass of spongy tissue full of blood vessels called the *placenta*, or afterbirth. This fastens itself to one side of the uterus, takes oxygen as well as nutriment from the mother and sends it through the umbilical cord to the child, the point of attachment being at the navel, the depression left on the belly of the child by the cutting of umbilical cord at birth. In the same way it takes the waste product from the child to the mother, and she in turn throws them out of her system through the kidneys, bowels and skin. The child and placenta are both encased within a membranous sac which secretes and serves to hold a watery fluid in which the child swims.

The child is folded together with legs on the thighs and thighs on the belly, arms on the chest and head bent forward over the breast. Toward the end of the term it moves about slightly, often stretches a little, and has periods of rest when it scarcely moves, and again periods of great activity. A mother first feels the child move in the fourth or fifth month. Often the young mother at this time begins to worry over her acts lest something she should do might deform the precious charge she carries. This, as you can readily understand from its early development, is impossible, for by the end of the second month the child has been formed, and no mental impressions of the mother can alter its shape. Just as the nucleus of the male sperm has within it all the contributions which the father of the child can give it, until after it is born, so does the mother give it its physical qualities right at the beginning.

Whatever is to be inherited from the father must be within the substance of the spermatozoon at the time the ovum is fertilized. He has no further pre-natal influence over it.

It is interesting to observe that the children of so-called great men are seldom above the average in intelligence, where, on the other hand, almost all men of great minds have had intelligent mothers.

How great or how little influence a mother has over her child through her thoughts has not been proven, nor has the subject of determining or influencing sex of the unborn child been settled.

At the end of nine months the child's development is complete and it is ready for its journey to the outside world. The process of this journey is called *labor*—a word which will describe the mother's share in it. When this occurs before the embryo is able to live outside the uterus it is known as *abortion*.

9 REPRODUCTION: HYGIENE OF PREGNANCY, MISCARRIAGE

In the previous chapter I said that if the process of labor occurs before the seventh month, which is the earliest time the *fetus* (or embryo) can live for any length of time outside the womb. It is known as *abortion* or *miscarriage*. When labor occurs later than this or within two weeks before term, it is known as *premature labor*.

The average girl in using the word abortion, has in mind a criminal act, whereby the process of pregnancy is purposely interrupted. She prefers the word *miscarriage*.

There is also the belief among girls that a miscarriage occurring in the early stages of pregnancy can be brought about without bad results or any serious consequences to her health.

It is a mistake to regard an abortion as of slight importance, for any interruption in the process of pregnancy is always more dangerous than the natural labor at full term. One writer claims there are more women ill in consequences of abortion than from full term childbirth, on account of which there are so many women who are semi-invalids.

There can be no doubt that the often excessive loss of blood leaves the girl in a weak and rundown condition thereby lessening her powers of resistance to other diseases.

The shock to the girl's system is greater than that produced by natural labor, and consequently leaves her in a hysterical and often critically nervous state for some time after.

The causes of abortion are many. Among them are overexertion, overexcitement, shock, fright, fall, great anger, dancing, fatigue, lifting heavy weights, purgative medicines and excessive sexual intercourse.

The dangers resulting from abortion are blood poison, hemorrhage—even lockjaw has been known to be the result of abortion, also the danger that one miscarriage is likely to follow another, and disables a woman to carry a child to the full term.

If there is the same care and treatment given the woman who aborts as the woman in childbirth, it will naturally be less likely to suffer serious results than if no medical attention were given her.

One of the most common disturbances of pregnancy is nausea, more commonly called "morning sickness," because it is felt in the morning when the woman first assumes the erect position. As a rule, this lasts only during the early months.

About the latter part of the fourth month, or often not before the fifth month, movements of the fetus are felt. These movements are called "life," and women are glad of this signal that all is progressing naturally. One writer said a woman had described the first feeling of life as "the trembling movements of a bird within my hand."

There are often many nervous manifestations accompanying the pregnant woman, such as headache, neuralgia, toothache and as a usual thing constipation is always present, and should receive attention. The teeth should also receive attention at this time for they decay easily on account of the secretions in the mouth which are increased during pregnancy.

The breasts enlarge in the early months of pregnancy, and there is a fullness and tingling felt often in the fifth week. The nipples become erect and the skin around the nipple becomes dark brown. These are only a few of the disturbances of pregnancy, but enough to show that other organs beside the uterus are tested in strength and how important it is to have a good healthy body. In fact, every tissue and fiber in the woman's body feels the impetus of pregnancy, and all kinds of physical changes occur.

One of the common questions asked by young women in early married life is how to tell if they are pregnant.

This is not always easy, but there are a few points on which a diagnosis is based, namely: in a healthy woman (during the reproductive age) the function of menstruation stops, together with morning sickness, and the enlargement of the breasts with dark color around the nipples, are early indications that pregnancy exists. I am not going to take the time nor space to explain that all three of the above named can exist in nervous women, even when pregnancy does not exist. It is, as I said earlier, with the average healthy girl I am dealing, not with the exception. The only certain signs of pregnancy are the hearing of the heart beats of the child and its movements.

Another question which troubles young women is how to count the time when she will be confined. This, too, is difficult to say, for an error of two weeks earlier or later is possible, because the time of conception is seldom definitely known. Experience has given a method of arriving at an approximate date which is used and which answers the purpose fairly well though it is by no means perfect. Add seven days to the first day of the last menstruation and count nine months forward. For example, Mrs. A menstruated last, beginning October 5; add seven days: this brings the date to October 12; add nine months, which brings the date of confinement to July 12. It is well to have every thing prepared two weeks before this date so that the woman can be as much as possible in the open air during the remaining waiting days.

The dress of the pregnant woman should receive serious attention. In the first place, it should be simple and warm, without bands restricting the circulation of any part of the body, like skirt bands, round garters, corsets and tight shoes. The secret of a comfortable outfit for the expectant mother is to have all clothing hang from the shoulders. Combination underwear can be bought as reasonably as the separate drawers and shirt. There should be no pressure on the womb from above, rather let all support come from below. The corset gets in its harmful work by pressing down the uterus into the pelvis, thus displacing the abdominal organs and crowding them together in such a way as to cause injury to the uterus as well as to the child itself. The muscles of the uterus and abdomen are weakened and from this results that horror of all women, "the high stomach." Some women, especially those having children, prefer to wear in the latter days of pregnancy an abdominal supporter. If it is well fitted to the body it helps to assist the abdominal muscles in carrying the weight and affords great relief. If women would devote to making themselves comfortable during pregnancy as much time as they give on the baby's outfit, they would profit by it. Instead of wearing any old worn out dress, ill fitting and out of style, make one "maternity" dress to fit the figure. This can, of course, be let out in size as the figure grows. It can be made of some pretty, inexpensive material and gives much comfort and ease to the mind as well as to the body that the woman who has once had one will never again do without one.

The food also should be simple. In fact, there are few restrictions to be placed on food unless so ordered by the physician. One common mistake of women is that they believe they are eating for two persons and, consequently, must gorge themselves, which, of course, results in indigestion. Physicians advise a small amount of meat once a day. Plenty of water, milk and cereals, fruit, vegetables and especially fruits, which loosens the bowels. Rich pastry or starches fried in fat should not be eaten, because they are hard to digest. There is no reason why the diet should be at all strict unless the woman is under the special care of a physician. She should take a moderate amount of exercise every day, but should not get tired. Walking in the open air in the sunlight is best. Avoid dancing, swimming and all violent exercise; sewing on the sewing machine should be restricted. Fainting in the early months is often caused from the bad air in overcrowded and overheated rooms, also from an empty stomach when the woman is too busy to notice nature's call for nourishment.

There is little more to be said here except that a pregnant woman should be mentally and physically active, though not fatigued. And of all things she should keep out of the hearing of old superstitions, which have a sign for every act and keep a young woman constantly worried. She should not be allowed to worry over her approaching labor, and as far as possible be kept cheerful and happy.

At the end of the period the child and the placenta are expelled from the uterus. The uterus gradually returns to its former size. It requires about six weeks for this to occur and it is very important that there should be no heavy lifting and overwork at this time. As a rule after childbirth the woman's form becomes matured and more developed. The facial expression takes on a kinder, a maternal look, the whole nervous system is awakened to sympathy, pain or grief bringing tears to the eyes quicker than ever before. Especially is this true for the first few years following.

The important thing is that the care of the pregnant woman should be begun in girlhood. If we are going to be and have mothers, then we should give attention to the development of the organs which make us mothers.

10 SOME CONSEQUENCES OF IGNORANCE AND SILENCE: CONTINENCE IN YOUNG MEN

When the boy arrives at the age of puberty, he is in greater danger than a girl of being not only led astray by companions, but being actually sent into unclean living by those nearest and most interested in his welfare—*his parents.*

The reason of this is that there has been and still is a false idea clinging to many parents that as soon as the boy has seminal emissions, it is a signal that he must have sexual relations or suffer in health.

That the seminal emissions are not harmful and that they grow less frequent as the boy grows older is a fact of which few mothers seem to be aware.

We cannot blame the mothers of the past for not informing their sons of this physical condition, for few of them knew it themselves. Mothers have been as ignorant as the boys of their sex functions as well as other functions of the body.

They accepted sickness, disease, and even death without a question, placing their faith and confidence entirely in the hands of the medical profession, who, like the rabbis and high priests made a church of their knowledge.

Fortunately this condition of affairs is changing, and the knowledge of the human body, which for ages has been most carefully locked within the medical libraries, is fast taking up its abode in the homes of the people—*where it belongs.*

It is said that in Japan the duty of a physician is to keep his patients in good health, receiving payment only when they are well.

Certainly this sounds like civilization.

Only a few weeks ago I had occasion to talk to a woman about her oldest son, whom I considered sick from overwork and lack of nourishment. She informed me, however, that this was not so, and whispered confidentially that he was 16 years old and "in that age when he needs a woman." She further remarked that she and "the papa" had talked it over with the result that the father had told the boy, when he had "the desire for a woman," that he, the father, "would give him money enough to get one."

Think of the boy's attitude toward women. Yet both parents had the sincerest wish to do their best for the boy; they gave the best advice they knew.

One of the most common errors I have found among people, even those educated in other lines of thought, is that the sexual organs will become useless unless they are used in early manhood. This is considered untrue by the best authorities on the subject, for it is known that the essential organs of reproduction are glands, not unlike the tear glands of the eyes or the milk glands of the breasts. The tear glands do not atrophy even if one does not cry for years, nor the milk glands during the entire period of reproduction. The same can be said of the sexual glands.

Another idea which is fast being uprooted is that the sexual act is an appetite, not unlike that of hunger or thirst, which must be fed by the boy sowing his "wild oats" first before settling down to marriage. It is now a recognized fact that it is no more necessary for a boy to "sow wild oats" than it is for a girl, and women are today demanding of men the same cleanliness of body and mind which men have heretofore considered necessary only in women.

It is now the unreserved opinion of the foremost medical men of the day that a man does not suffer in health from living a continent life, not is he a "mollycoddle" from so doing.

Hutchinson says: "The belief that the exercise of the sex functions is necessary to the health of the male at any age is a pure delusion, while before full maturity it is highly injurious."

Ruggles says: "Sexual abstinence is compatible with perfect health and tends to increase virility (which means manhood) through the reabsorption of the semen."

The ancient Teutons were aware of this for it is said

that it was considered a most shameful thing for their young men to have sexual relations with a woman before his twenty-sixth year. From observation and experience they were convinced that men were not sexually mature much before this age, and no one will dispute they were strong and manly.

Statistics show that 65 percent of men infected with venereal diseases (which means diseases due to sexual intercourse) are contracted between the ages of 15 and 21 years; and 25 percent are contracted in the 21st and 23rd years.

Many writers claim that from statistics they have found men are not sexually mature before the twenty-fifth year, and women not before the twentieth year. Yet we find them both reeking with sexual diseases before this age.

According to Sanger's *History of Prostitution*, it is claimed that three-eighths of the prostitutes enter the life before the twentieth year in New York City. It is safe to say this is a conservative estimate, for the more recent investigations in Chicago and other cities show a very much higher percentage. However, this, together with the statistics of venereal diseases mentioned above, show that it is before the boy and girl are sexually mature, that there is the greatest difficulty in directing the impulses and controlling the passions.

Chassaignac says that the more healthy and normal an individual is, the better can he not only control his passions, but the less likely is he to be disturbed by continence.

Just one more word on the subject of continence, and that is that it is not at all unusual to find men determined to remain continent until they find their ideal woman. Nor for athletes in training engaged in contests, nor for sailors on long sea voyages, and many others for long periods of time is continence impossible; in fact, they are the better for it.

This knowledge was not lost sight of in ancient times. Reference is made to it in the Bible, in the sending of women prostitutes into the camps of the enemy the night before an expected battle, in order to exhaust or decease the vitality of the soldiers.

When one finds an individual who realizes the force of the sexual impulses and knows how to conserve them, you usually find a person who does not drain or exhaust these forces, but uses them in bigger work.

Every girl should look upon the man who indulges freely in the sexual relations as a creature *without social responsibility*, as a prostitute far more degraded than the unfortunate girl who is compelled to sell her body to sustain life.

Every girl should know something about the physical makeup of a boy as well as of her own, for upon the well being of both does the future of the race depend. To be a real mother, a woman must understand a boy's emotions and development, if she would sympathize with him. And when she does understand, she will not send him to buy a woman for physical satisfaction.

It is the ignorance of parents together with the silence of the medical profession, which is largely responsible for the terrible spread of venereal diseases which exists today.

When a few years ago Dr. Morrow stated that there is more venereal diseases among innocent virtuous wives, than among prostitutes, this statement should have resounded throughout the walls of every home in the land, instead of which it is kept intact within the covers of large volumes, where only those wearing cap and gown have access to it.

It is claimed that out of 1,000 married men in New York, 800 have gonorrhea, and 90 percent of these have not been cured and can infect their wives. The result is that at least three out of every five married women in New York have gonorrhea.

This seems astounding and exaggerated, but the following quotation is taken from an authority and is considered quite conservative: "Over 90 percent of our young men stray from the path of virtue before marriage; 60 percent contract venereal diseases which are difficult to cure; more wives than prostitutes have venereal diseases; one-eighth of all diseases in New York hospitals are venereal; 20,000 infected persons walk the streets daily."

It seems to me that the above facts are sufficient to warrant every girl and boy knowing something about these diseases.

11 SOME CONSEQUENCES OF IGNORANCE AND SILENCE: GONORRHEA

The two venereal diseases which I will tell you something of here are those most commonly known to all, gonorrhea and syphilis.

Gonorrhea is an inflammation of the urethra (water passage) characterized by redness, swelling, smarting pain on the passing of water, and accompanied by a thick purulent (poisonous) discharge, at first creamy in color, and later a greenish yellow. It is considered by the highest authorities as solely a sexual disease in adults, depending almost exclusively upon sexual intercourse as its mode of origin and infection. In children, however, it is not the rule, especially in infants and little girls, who can be infected by the hands of the mother or nurse being soiled with the discharge, also where the fresh discharge is on towels, toilets, etc. It starts as an inflammation of the outer delicate parts but seldom enters the urethra.

In former days gonorrhea was considered an ordinary catarrhal inflammation, "no worse than a bad cold," the old saying went. It was thought to originate in women with the discharge at the end of the menstrual period, or leucorrhoea; in fact, any secretions from the uterus, of an irritating character, were thought to be sources of gonorrhea. However, with the discovery of the microbe "gonococcus," in 1879, by Dr. Neisser, it is now an established fact that the disease comes from a source where there is either latent or chronic gonorrhea, which of course, means that the gonococcus is present. It is considered a conservative estimate that at least 50 percent of the adult population in this country have suffered from gonococca infection. More men than women have been and are infected.

The first symptoms of the disease appear from three to seven days after infection, and under proper treatment the discharge may disappear in six or eight weeks.

If the man or woman places himself under the care of a specialist within forty-eight hours after infection, the disease is often of much shorter duration. When allowed to become chronic, it is called *gleet*. Too much emphasis cannot be out upon the danger of placing any one with the disease into the hands of doctors who advertise so conspicuously, claiming rapid and complete cures for all sexual diseases. Experience has found that thousands of boys and young men, attracted by such alluring promises as only the quack can put forth, have been under such treatment, only to find later that the disease was allowed to remain in the tissues, the discharge only having been dried up. The germs were allowed to continue their work on up into the bladder, kidneys, joints, heart and even to the brain. The germs can live for years in the body hidden away in the gland ducts, the mucous membrane of the organ first attacked being in a normal state, yet when a condition arises when the vitality of the tissues in which the germs are lodged is lowered, or which gives the germs themselves more nourishment or stimulus, such as alcohol or excessive intercourse, they almost always become active again.

In women the small part of the womb (cervix), as well as the urethra, are favorite places of attack. When the disease attacks the cervix a woman may not be conscious of it, and so, unless prominent symptoms attend it, she may infect many persons in the meantime. In man, on the other hand, the disease cannot be present without his knowing there is something wrong, and it should be impressed upon him that it is a moral obligation on his part not to have sexual relations until he has been examined and pronounced cured by a specialist in genitourinary diseases.

Your general practitioner will always recommend to you a specialist if you ask him to. When the disease attacks the uterus and ovaries it very often blocks the fallopian tubes and prevents the impregnation of the ovum. It is said that over one-third of the childless marriages are due to gonorrhea in women innocently contracted from their husbands. Both men and women can become sterile from this disease. The seminal tubes in the man become blocked, thus disabling him from impregnating the ovum.

Again, when the disease attacks the organs of generation, unless speedily attended to, the organs get into a chronic state of inflammation. They are therefore more difficult to reach, the chances of cure more difficult, and it usually means an operation for the woman.

The great mass of ailing women who trace their misery back to never seeing a well day since marriage, can be classed among those suffering with this disease, as can also that army of women whose illness is classed among "female disorders."

A curious point to know is that a man may have a hidden or latent gonorrhea, infect a clean, healthy woman during the sexual relations, and she, in turn, can infect him with the same disease. The great majority of infections in women are contracted from men who believe themselves cured, being under the false impression that they are cured because the discharge has ceased.

At a lecture given by a well-known physician in this city last winter, the physician advised every girl whose sweetheart, lover, or expected husband had a history of inflammatory rheumatism of the joints back of him, that as she valued her life and future health, not to marry that man without a thorough examination by a specialist in these diseases. He declared: no young man should have inflammatory rheumatism. This statement is considered somewhat exaggerated by some making more recent investigations, yet all seem to agree that a very large majority of cases of inflammatory rheumatism of the joints have the gonococcus present.

If the woman is not made sterile by the disease and is able to carry the child to full term labor, then there is another danger of infecting the child's eyes during the process of labor, when the secretions lodge themselves into the delicate membrane of the eyes. Then, unless quick action is applied, the sight of both eyes can be lost. Over 80 percent of blindness in babies is due to this germ. It can be carried into the eyes of both children and adults by any means which can carry the discharge to the eyes. Upon the slightest suspicion that this has been done, medical aid should be summoned at once.

There is one fortunate thing to know , that the germ cannot live for a great length of time outside its natural or proper environment , though it can for years be hidden in the body. It dries up very quickly, and special solutions of both bichloride and permanganate of potash will kill the germs with which the solutions come in contact. There is but one course to follow, that upon any of the symptoms mentioned above, go at once to a reliable physician and follow his instructions closely. And remember that the causes which retard recovery are alcoholic drinks, lack of rest, spicy food and *sexual excitement*. It is said there is no positive proof against this disease, except continency until marriage and then monogamy.

That both the United States army and navy give out special instructions to the soldiers and sailors to enable them to avoid infection so far as possible is now generally known.

A story is told of a young Irish physician, who, being

asked how he treated gonorrhea, replied most tersely, "with contempt." That this was for a time a general feeling is agreed, but with the knowledge that so many persons, especially women, contract the disease under the moral, as well as legal, conditions of present society, the feeling has changed. A woman is infected by her husband after the marriage is sanctioned by the state and blessed by the church, neither taking the interest in the woman's future to guarantee to her a clean individual as a husband. Prostitution has been upheld and women segregated for man's sexual use, the government going to the extent of authorizing examinations of the women for venereal diseases to insure *man's* safety from these diseases. Yet there has been no such protection given either the woman prostitute or the wife that the man's body is free from them. On the other hand, every means to keep a married woman in ignorance of the source of her infection is made by church, state and society in general. Every law to protect the man's crime is made for his use, while women remain unprotected victims of his guilt. And this, they say, is "to protect the family and the home!"

Dr. James S. Wood tells a story of his experience with a young woman of 25, married five years, when she came to him. The husband admitted having had gonorrhea previous to marriage. The doctor found her flowing excessively, the cervix badly torn, the uterus sharply bent back and fixed, ovaries bound down and adherent, the tubes thickened; a leucorrheal discharge was present which contained gonococci, and other symptoms which made her sick and miserable. The doctor operated upon her, scraping her womb, sewing the torn cervix, opening the abdomen to remove the thickened appendix and inflamed ovaries and tubes. She convalesced beautifully, and had no bad or unusual symptoms for six months, at which time she returned with a renewed infection. Careful questioning extracted from the husband the confession that he had been "out with the boys," and had had a recurrence of gonorrhea. Most of the good which came from the operation was spoiled by this second infection.

This is only one simple example of what is meant by preserving the home and family at the terrible cost of women's lives. Women should protest against the so-called medical secret which decrees that they be kept in ignorance where their health, as well as life, is directly concerned. That there are men in the medical profession in this country, as well as in Europe, who have openly protested against respecting the secret where another life is involved, seems a cheerful signal of a general social awakening in this field.

In the *Medical Record*, April 20, 1912, Maude Glasgow says: "After suffering for years a woman becomes a feeble, worn-out, nervous wreck: her life is a burden. The operating table is her only hope and she leaves it deformed, mutilated and sexless."

If women voluntarily exposed themselves to diseases which would sap the husband's vitality, making him a dependent invalid, or expose him to the shock of a mutilating operation or death—would men continue to suffer? Would they allow the medical secret to protect women in this alleged "freedom"? Every girl knows he would neither protect her nor continue to suffer. It is women only who have allowed the double standard of morals to stand so long, giving men the purest and best of their womanhood, but not demanding the same from them. As soon as women realize the danger to themselves and their children which they are likely to incur from men who have lived promiscuously, they will revolt against such standards.

Gonorrhea differs from syphilis, and though it is not a disease which can be transmitted from the parent to the children, as syphilis can, yet it is a subtle, wrecking disease and can do almost as much harm to the individual.

12 SOME CONSEQUENCES OF IGNORANCE AND SILENCE: SYPHILIS

Prominent medical authorities claim that syphilis was not known in Europe before the discovery of America. Others equally as prominent hold that it has existed for many centuries in Europe, but was confused with other diseased such as leprosy. It makes little difference to the girl or boy today just how long or where it came from; the point we do know is that it is here in our homes and workshops, and we should know what it is like and how to avoid it.

A story is told of a French nobleman whose son was about to leave his home to live in a big city. Said the father to the son: "If you are not afraid of God, fear at least syphilis." This advice might be applied today, for if boys or girls knew, or could see the appalling results of syphilis, they would surely fear it, for it is humanity's most deadly foe.

Syphilis is an infectious disease, caused by a special microbe which is acquired by contagion or heredity.

It is chronic in course, varied and intermittent in character, and the length of time it remains in the body is indefinite.

It is so widespread that no country in the world is free from it, neither is any organ of the body exempt from its ravages.

Let us take a young man accustomed to promiscuous sexual intercourse, who cohabits with a syphilitic woman. He notices nothing wrong for about five weeks, when he becomes aware of a pimple on the sexual organs to which perhaps he pays little attention. This grows and becomes hard at the base and ulcerated on the top.

About ten days after the appearance of the ulcer (or chancre) the boy notices that the glands of the groins begin to swell, but as there is little or no pain attached he still pays no attention to all this.

After three, or sometimes four, weeks the ulcerated opening heals, but leaves the hard lump under the skin. In two or even three months after the time of infection the first general symptoms appear. His bones ache, he is mentally depressed, slightly feverish at night, and a rash appears upon his body and sore spots in the mouth. These symptoms usually decide him to consult a doctor, who finds him in the second stage of syphilis. This condition lasts usually about two and a half years, the rash often lasting a short period, and leaving, but to return again.

The blood and ulcers on the body contain the poisons of the disease, and for three or four years the poison *can be transmitted* by contagion, or by heredity.

The third stage is the most destructive, especially to the nervous system, for this disease is recognized as the greatest factor in organic disturbances of the nervous system.

It not rarely is the cause of cerebral and spinal meningitis, paralysis of the legs, paralysis of one side of the body, and that most helpless and terrible disease, softening of the brain, and many other diseases which affect the spinal cord and which are seldom ever cured. The majority of those diseased are left with physical or mental infirmities, rendering them public charges.

There have been cases where the third stage did not develop and as this stage is not distinctly separated from the second stage by a definite line, it may not take place for months, or even years after the first sore appeared. Again, this stage has been averted by careful treatment in the early stages, and it is here the hope of all afflicted lies.

Every case of syphilis begins with the characteristic pimple or chancre, except inherited syphilis. The chancre always appears where the infection enters, and the glands swell in the same vicinity. For instance, if in using a pipe of a syphilitic, whose mouth contains the sore patches, the victim finds the chancre will appear on his lips, mouth, or throat, and the glands of the neck will swell.

It is said that almost 10 percent of the infections are contracted innocently, especially in European countries, where kissing and other forms of endearment are much indulged in. In this country it is not so common, but more women than men contract it innocently and in this manner.

In women, too, the first symptoms are not so characteristic as in men. She may pay no attention to the chancre for a month, even if she does feel aches in the bones, she thinks she is run down, or thinks she has malaria; even the rash does not alarm her, and often only repeated miscarriages will be the only symptoms she can remember of the early stages. She may continue for years before the disease reaches the third stage. This is not always so, for in every individual the disease differs in character and duration.

Gonorrhea and syphilis differ in many ways. For instance, the former shows itself in a week or ten days after infection, where syphilis shows no signs for five or six weeks.

Gonorrhea is considered a purely sexual disease, because infection takes place only in sexual relations (except where the germ gets into the eyes), while syphilis can be contracted in many other ways, through forks, spoons, glasses or cups, towels, sponges, bathtubs, toilets, pipes, dental and barbers' instruments and kissing.

Gonorrhea is considered a social danger because of its effect upon the sexual organs, often rendering them sterile. Syphilis is also a social danger, but it has a direct effect upon the offspring, and upon future generations because its effects are visited upon the child.

Sixty to 80 percent of the syphilitic offspring die at birth or in early infancy. Someone has well said, "The greater criminal is he who poisons the germ cells."

In hereditary syphilis there is more difficulty in gathering facts, for the laws which control it are not so well understood, as yet.

There is no sore or chancre in hereditary syphilis but other symptoms appear which every physician recognizes and of course attends to at birth.

Under proper treatment the danger of the father transmitting the disease to the child should cease in from two to five years, while the danger of the mother transmitting it to her offspring does not end at any definite time.

There have been mothers known to have given birth to syphilitic offspring years after all disappearance of their own symptoms.

The strongest features of the disease transmitted to the offspring are the deformities which it imparts to the bones of the head as well as of the body.

It is said on good authority that if a patient, at the end of five years, has been two years without symptoms of treatment, he may be guaranteed for marriage. Though he can never be wholly guaranteed from relapses in his own person. These however, are considered noninfectious.

The cure of the disease depends upon the individual's environment, constitution and his habits, chiefly as regards alcohol and tobacco.

Alcohol is considered the commonest and most active enemy of the patient's recovery. Men addicted to the use of alcohol are the most difficult to cure.

There seems to be no doubt that if the disease receives the proper treatment there is every hope of the individual to live a normal life. Fournier, a French authority, says:

"Personally I could cite several hundred observations concerning syphilitic subjects who, after undergoing thorough treatment, have married and became fathers of healthy, good-looking children." The question, then, to receive some attention is what means are valuable for the treatment of both syphilis and gonorrhea.

Dr. Prince A. Morrow says: "Prompt curative treatment is not only in the interests of the patients themselves, but especially in the interests of the others they might infect. But everywhere we are confronted with this situation: There are no special hospitals for this class of diseases; few general hospitals receive them in the early, curable stage; still fewer have special venereal wards; even the dispensary services are not organized with special adaptation to the needs of venereal cases; few have night classes, so that working people who go to the dispensary must lose half a day, which often means the sacrifice of their employment. As a consequence they resort to quacks or the use of nostrums (secret or quack medicines). They are not cured, but go on spreading the seeds of contagion."

This is the condition as far as hospitals are concerned in the matter of venereal diseases. And in the relation to private practice the average person's position is still more deplorable. Take, for example, the story of a girl who came under my care some years ago, after having suffered three years with the disease. She had been refused attendance in public hospitals in three different cities while she was working her way to New York. At different times she consulted physicians, only to learn that to be cured she must be treated regularly, and to be so treated would require money. Different estimates were quoted her from $150 to $500 for treatment. As the amount of money left over after she had paid her expenses each week was never over $2, the possibility of a cure looked hopeless. She concluded to purchase patent medicines whenever she could, but her condition became worse, until she was picked up by a charitable organization, who cared for her until she died. When I saw her all hair; eyebrows and eyelashes were gone, her nose and upper lip were eaten almost entirely away, most of her teeth were gone—in fact, to try to describe her condition would be almost impossible.

This is only one case, but there are thousands of syphilitics who are wandering about unable to pay the prices which the physician asks to treat this disease. The same can be said of gonorrhea, and the same physician who clamors against the prices of the so-called quack, forgets that the price he asks of the public is exorbitant in the extreme. So the only course for the individual to take, if he cannot pay the price, is to remain a menace to society. The physician assumes no responsibility toward society to find out if the patient is under treatment elsewhere; the patient can do as he pleases with his disease when he closes the doctor's door. This, then, is the situation as regard society's attitude toward the venereal subject: Society seems to take a different attitude towards other contagious and infectious diseases, such as measles, chickenpox, diphtheria, etc. In these diseases, a physician has some responsibility towards society, he must report each case as it comes to his attention, to the Board of Health, who in turn assumes some responsibility by isolating the disease.

If this is necessary in these comparatively simple diseases, how much more important should it be to register and isolate patients suffering from the venereal diseases.

13 MENOPAUSE

In the chapter on Puberty, it was stated that the menstrual function began in the average girl at fifteen years of age and continued until the 45th or 50th year.

At this later age it ceases, together with her sexual or childbearing capabilities and is known as Menopause or Change of Life.

This constitutes a period from the beginning of irregularities in the appearance of the menstrual flow, until it has actually ceased, which period usually lasts two and one-half to three years.

Thousands of women know nothing of the period which, like puberty, they must pass through, but are entirely ignorant of the process.

It is usual for them to look toward this age with dread and foreboding; where a little knowledge of the nature of the process would enable them to enter upon this period physically prepared, which would insure their safe arrival through this dreaded and much-feared period.

The greatest change occurring in the woman at this time is that which goes on in the ovaries. They cease to do their work and ovulation stops.

The first indication that the woman has, that this is likely to occur, is by the ceasing of the menses or monthlies.

Ovulation, however, very often continues for several months, even a year after menstruation has entirely ceased.

The glandular tissues of the uterus, tubes and ovaries degenerate, which is said to account for the Menopause, and that of the ovaries occurs later than the tubes and uterus, which explains the continuance of ovulation after the menses have stopped.

In a few women the Menopause is accompanied by very little or almost no discomfort at all, just a sudden stopping of the monthlies announces to them that this period has come.

The majority, however, do not pass through this tie so easily, but suffer for the entire period with one affliction or another.

Among those symptoms most common are flushings or flashes, which are mostly confined to head, face and neck, are increased by heat and motion and followed by profuse sweating, giddiness, backache, headache, sleeplessness, disturbances of digestion like diarrhea or constipation, blueness, depression of spirits, shortness of breath, palpitation and nervous irritability.

But the most alarming symptom of the Menopause is

hemorrhage. This is too often considered lightly and classed with the minor symptoms of this period.

Whenever there is excessive bleeding, there is surely a cause and calls for special and immediate attention. It may be caused by an inflamed condition of the lining of the uterus (womb); ulceration, general diseases of the heart, lungs and kidneys can also be the cause of excessive bleeding at this period. Some authorities claim that it also has its cause in early or profuse menstruation, too frequent and difficult labors, abortions and alcoholic drinking, but the most common cause of hemorrhage at this time is cancer. It is a fact that cancer in women, from the age of 40 to 50 is more common that at any other age.

Perhaps it is not generally known that cancer is now known to begin as a local disease, and if taken in time it can be removed so completely that radical cure follows. No wonder then, that hemorrhage should be an alarming symptom, for if care is not taken and the dreaded disease, cancer, is allowed to take root, the results are too generally known to dwell upon. At the first signs of hemorrhages or excessive flow, a woman should place herself under the care of a gynecologist (specialist in the diseases of woman), just as a pregnant woman is under the care of a physician until she is entirely free from the dangers of childbirth.

Women have heretofore looked to this period with dread, on account of the consequences which neglect has caused. It need not be dreaded for assuring word comes from prominent physicians who have made this special period a study, that the natural symptoms of the Menopause do not portent loss of life, reason or health. It is a period as natural to the woman as menstruation and with little care, these symptoms or ailments will cease in a few years, leaving the woman to enjoy years of good health.

When the period is delayed beyond the fiftieth year, it calls for the same attention as excessive flow. These are two important signs of disease, and should receive immediate care. The period is, however, often brought about at an earlier age than is normal, by mental or physical shock, illness, operations, etc.

The age at which it occurs often differs with climate, race and, according to Kisch, social relations, who claims, that the sexual function is "generally abolished earlier in the laboring classes, who are compelled to work hard and have many cares," and further states that a vigorous vitality causes prolongation of the menstrual process.

In the average woman it does not cease at once, but has two or three periods of cessation, returns again for an irregular period and continues in this irregularity for the entire time of two and one-half to three years. It is important to know that the changes which are going on in the organs of the woman are exactly opposite from those which occur at puberty.

At puberty the organs are increasing with life, vigor, and vitality, white at the Menopause they are receding or going backward.

The generative organs gradually but surely shrink or atrophy after menstruation stops. The uterus becomes small. The vagina, whose walls were formerly corrugated or wrinkled, now become smooth. The orifice or opening of the vagina, becomes shrunken, unless it has been previously enlarged by child-bearing. The whole process tends to show that the childbearing period is at end, which in fact has caused much mental anxiety and disturbance among women to the extent of melancholy and insanity.

It seems a very small thing to give to every woman, going through this disagreeable period of life—a complete change of climate and rest, until the change has become established. Certainly she has served society to the best of her knowledge, often "entering into the valley of the shadow of death"; many times fearlessly, to give the best of herself to the race. It is a small thing to give in return.

All that is needed is to keep guard on oneself—watch the diet and bowels. A light vegetable diet seems best at this time unless very actively engaged in physical exercise, then meat once a day. Keep free from foods difficult to digest, cheese, fried foods, hot bread, etc., drink plenty of water and eat fruit to keep the bowels open; slight exercise in the open air, rest, sleep and freedom from mental anxiety are the simple rules which are generally prescribed for women at this stage of their lives.

14 CONCLUSION

In conclusion, I cannot refrain front saying that women must come to recognize there is some function of womanhood other than being a childbearing machine. Too long have they allowed themselves to become this, bowing to the yoke of motherhood from puberty to the grave. No other thought has entered the mind except to be a good mother—which has usually meant a slave-mother. This has been her only use, her only wish and hope—and when the age arrives where she cannot perform this function longer, she considers herself useless. No wonder she becomes melancholic or even insane.

Fortunately the woman of today is gradually ridding herself of such archaic notions. More and more is she realizing that motherhood is only one of her capabilities; that there are certain individuals more fitted for mother-hood that others, just as individuals are better fitted for nursing, teaching, etc.

And further must she realize that though she is past the age of motherhood, yet she is still a woman with all the instincts and experiences which motherhood has bestowed upon her, and she can now begin a new development, based upon these valuable experiences, she can now enter into public life unhampered by the details of kitchen and babies, for as she completes her work and passes on, others come in to take her place.

Being free from domestic and maternal cares enables her to give to society the benefit of her matured thought, seasoned and enriched by these experiences.

She often does enjoy the best health of her life after the Menopause and this, together with a vista of a future of usefulness, should open to the woman in the post-climacteric period, a new life—a new world.

I cannot refrain from uttering just a word about the relation of the entire subject I have been discussing to the economic problem. It is impossible to separate the ignorance of parents, prostitution, venereal diseases, or the silence of the medical profession from the great economic questions that the world is facing today. It is here ever before us, and the more we look into the so-called evils of the day the more we realize that the whole structure of the present day society is built upon a rotten and decaying foundation. Until capitalism is swept away, there is no hope for young girls to live a beautiful life during their girlhood. There is no hope for boys or girls to build up strong and sturdy bodies. There is no hope that a woman can live in the family relation and have children without sacrificing every vestige of individual development. There is no hope that prostitution will cease, as long as there is hunger. There is no hope for a strong race as long as venereal diseases exist. And they will exist until women rise in one big sisterhood to fight this capitalist society which compels a woman to serve as a sex implement for man's use.

Education is necessary—education is the need of the people. For this will soon enable one to see that knowledge alone does not suffice, but that it is only through economic security that the man and the woman will emerge in a future civilization.

ABOUT THE AUTHOR

Margaret Sanger (1879–1966) was a nurse, sex educator and birth control activist. In 1916 she opened the first birth control clinic in the U.S.; soon after, she was arrested and jailed for distributing contraceptives. She founded the American Birth Control League in 1921 and became the first president of the International Planned Parenthood Federation in 1953. Other works include *What Every Mother Should Know, The Case of Birth Control* and *An Autobiography.*

9 781518 749483

www.ingramcontent.com/pod-product-compliance
Lightning Source LLC
Chambersburg PA
CBHW062015280526
45787CB00005B/2103